Comforting

THE DIABETIC HEART

**A PERSONAL STORY OF THE GOOD LIFE
FIFTY YEARS WITH DIABETES**

Toliendo

Title: Comforting The Diabetic Heart
Copyright©2020 Teo Tioliendo

Publisher: Twinteum Publishing Company
Twintium Inc.
schenariandesword@gmail.com

All Rights Reserved. No Part of this book may be reproduced, reprinted, stored in electronic retrieval system, or transmitted by any means, electronic, mechanical, by video, online, photocopying, or otherwise without written permission of Artist, Teo Tioliendo, or Twinteum Inc.

Cover Art Title* 'Comforting The Diabetic Heart' Tioliendo
Art Copyright ©2020 Teo Tioliendo
ISBN: 9798605425847
Printed Edition
Printed in the United States

"Are you ready to eat yet?" His father had been a diabetic fifty years. In all those years taking care of himself on his own, accepting his lifestyle as a diabetic, using his southern chef style of cooking to enjoy his food, he never once mentioned fasting. But did fast, he just didn't call it fasting. He said he wasn't hungry yet. In this way, each morning, he put off eating, instead of doing by habit he used to do, just after he was awake, and that was to eat a southern breakfast. In this way he fasted. He did well after that. When he, at last, ate, eating was then a comfort to his heart.

A Comfort To The Heart

Centered at the heart of this story of a person, a man, a father, a diabetic, is learning to see that the most important focus in a person's experiences with diabetes, was what a son learned from taking care of his diabetic father the last 15 years of his life, is what his son learned about the importance of caring for and comforting the diabetic heart. The son stood over his father when he took his last breath, and at that moment the Holy Spirit washed the son's heart clean of a lifetime of bitterness, anger, sorrow, sadness, heaviness, fear, and feeling of pain from being outcast by his family and siblings all his life, who pretended it was otherwise. His father's prayers for his son, at the moment of his passing, were answered and had brought his son a blessing, a benediction, that remove all these things from his heart. Something went inside him and healed his heart, his mind, and gave him a new start with his family, though they would never change and continued the same treatment of him as they had done all through the years. Still, the son was hanged, and the past never affected him the same again. Then the day came he, the son had become diabetic, but he learned a lot from his father, from caring for him, working with him to control, treat, endure the sacrifice that come with caring for a diabetic, and he sought to help his family, regardless of their sins against him, sins of not caring, and sin of not listening. When you become diabetic you now have a diabetic heart that needs you to focus on your heart for longevity and a good life. Diabetic's experiencing the appearance of nothing going on with their heart might need to look again and make a covenant with themselves to be faithful to the health of their heart. Diabetes was the beginning of a new heart life. The son had been a student of the study of life which is philosophy, at the university, but he lived by common sense. He had learned from school to form a question in his mind and then too find the answer to that question. How is my heart, and why is it beating, s hard, so fast every time I eat? He learned to pay attention to the speed of his heart, after eating. It's beating. It was an important lesson he learned, and taught himself. "You have to keep listening to yourself, to your heart. Slow heartbeat, fast heartbeat, signs of how food is affecting your heart's beating. Can you hear and feel where your heart is steady, struggling, in a palpitation, or smooth with comfortable beats. Stories of people dying suddenly of heart attacks from diabetes, actually diabetic heats, scared the young man. A syrup from a cup of hot chocolate, too much cinnamon, caffeine in chocolate, had never cause palpitations before, or so you thought until now, that is now you are diabetic, looking to reverse your diabetes. But then you realize you had been having palpitations, getting EKGs over and over in the past for years, cause of your sudden attack of heart beat run wild; for reason the EKG did not reveal. Never heard of too much sugar in your blood, (ketoacidosis) the need for good cholesterol, nearly having a heart attack during sex, loss of blood flow to keep virile, the possibility of potency, the whole body system is attack, but *Tumeric* addresses the whole body system that is affected by diabetes, high sugar. Breathing became a thing to lower blood pressure. Meditation and breathing had helped him over twenty years in the martial arts, now it revealed its power to help the blood, again something that he knew but never consciously thought about, just did, in the past. But sugar introduced him to diabetic relevant words, terms, and abilities of his complex body's, natural abilities, that help the body quickly when needed. The damage he did to himself by eating, drinking, because it was convenient, fast, quick, tasty, and pleasurable, over working, lacking in nutrients, balance worked against his health, kept his sugar imbalanced, high and low, never at perfect sugar balance to the harm of his body, but especially his heart. He did not approach the sugar problem he had the way he helped his Dad. He did what his father wanted him to do according to the instructions of his doctors. He took care of his sugar that way at first, then he heard how insulin ended in blowing out a diabetic's kidneys. He never took pills, medicines, and he wanted to get back to his natural approach to healing. Pills, insulin, were for emergencies, blockers, controllers, not cures. He had looked for the cures and that had never ended. The question he asked since he was nineteen, he still asked himself. "Is there a cure for diabetes and Alzheimer's, the two diseases killing of our family for years and years in later years?" He put the question to today's artificial intelligence information source. He began to piece together needs of the body and the problems and the approach to hit the all at once. The answer came in the form of a process that is mentioned above, for him. Spices, fasting, low carbs, fruits and vegetables, it was what Dad ate. What he did. But Dad could not read for years, and would never have known what I learned on his own. He had never read the Bible to his son. He grew up I the church though, the son's mother had told him. His father never used turmeric, *korkum*, (*sapphron*) in Hebrew, in the Bible, that had helped his son reverse his diabetes, and attain excellent sugar balance, and helped him to begin a new chapter of life with the natural cure for diabetes, as a type 2 diabetic. A day at a time cure. All the ideas of many scientist and doctors, their treatments, cures, programs, diets, helped the body. Carbs and proteins must be understood for their benefits and how they help and harm the sugar's balance. The natural power of the body was again the most reliable when using the lifestyle tailored for the particular diabetic's cure as it worked for the individual and diabetics. What happened to make these generational diseases so wide spread? "Additives." Additive stocks are still thirty years strong, and even sold on the stock exchange. The son became diabetic from juices, teas, ice cream with "Corn syrup" the rumor was in his family, and when he stopped walking eight miles a day, making 620 deliveries a day. Burning off the two quarts of juice, sugar loaded, at work all the time had become his norm. Juice and teas he drank for energy left his heart beat slow, his mind depressed, his energy quickly turned to exhaustion, tiredness. The body pain, chronic inflammation, palpitations, he still believed he was being healthy by drinking his juices. He drank juices at home, after eating, during a day's activities, or before sleeping or resting, while rejuvenating in inactivity. Low blood sugar, high blood sugar, the whole experience of diabetes is a whole body experience, after all, because blood travels through the heart, through the whole body system. He later learned the juices with the additives ruin his health regardless of what he thought was a healthy lifestyle. The Word of God told us life is in the blood. Where your blood sugar has gone is the result of disease causing foods, or good food. The son asked himself, "What lying spirits are at work influencing the unhealthy activities that have caused you to become a diabetic?" There are genetic factors, but people have genetic factors all their life, but don't switch on to being diabetics. But additives ignore the genetic when you consume, eat, additives, to directly activate insulin over production to lead to insulin resistance, to diabetes. Japan is even plague "Who knew they had some many elders with cancer because of their additives. Why would anybody eat foods that cause generational diseases such as diabetes and Alzheimer's? Poverty, eating the sweet poisons of cheap foods, not knowing the science, lying spirits behind food providers feeding the world? Even pantry foods have these generational disease causing food additives, "linked to" diabetes and Alzheimers. Additives have made millions, billions, while causing diseases. The son eliminated all additives from his diet and the true healing took hold. His discipline of the new life, that is the new lifestyle, and a healthy, claer, strengthened heart. So he was comforted as he looked forward for what was to come from the reversal of his lifestyle that leads to diabetes. What hits the whole body system to heal the body, in contrast to, the whole body damaging effect that diabetes could cause, was for the son, he knowledge of the healing abilities of the many parts of what make up the process, lifestyle of a cure for this generational disease. Tumeric, the knowledge of the healing of the nerves, virus killing herbs, (gingko, gensing) an spices that heals the whole body system, apple cider vinegar to cleanse, care for diabetic feet, healing foods for nerves, protecting your eyes from blindness, olive oil, beets, garlic, sauerkraut, heart attacks, rashes, apple cider vinegar for feet, stopping, cracks, infections, fungus infections, reversing cortisol weight gain, all these the son had learned were never even spoken of the years he cared for his diabetic father. But when he became diabetic he had mastered and learned to prevent the same fate that was his father's diabetic lifestyle. He used fasting, turmeric (with black pepper), being fortunate not to be able to have Sulphur in his foods. So he listens to his heart beats, and comforts his heart by eating well, which comes with healing. The fifty years his father was diabetic were great the first 35 years. He could have gone on dialysis and lives longer. He at the last moment felt his heart stop, he knew by his expression, but a week later he still felt the gift from God sent to him from heaven, and the inspiration that continues from caring for him and learning from the way he lived with his   diabetes that few people realize was always about the   diabetic's   greatest   challenge, comforting the diabetic heart. God put spices in nature to help with this whole body system problem. A diabetic must, learn how to take care of their diabetic heart.

This is where this story begins how a country boy a young father's diabetic life, came to the comfort of his heart, after living with diabetes nearly his whole life, life across fifty years of being a diabetic. This was just before medicine returned to right foods, and the spices in organic nature, for approaches to cures that medicines are not able to provide without medicines that are paradoxically insulin causes for diabetes and insulin controls for insulin, in contradiction to how spices naturally help balance sugar levels without insulin for insulin paradoxical experiences that the father's son was able to use to free himself from the whole system challenges to be healthy as a diabetic. The diabetic father's experience was to catch up to this new understanding. His life before, is his story, being told here, and what generations of diabetics were to learn from him. What is in a man's heart, this cannot be told by having a diabetic heart, but it is a comfort to the heart to know you can live with a diabetic heart, for all the comforts there are in life for a healthy heart to be beat strong.

A Diabetic For Fifty Years

A Diabetic Father For Fifty Years A father became a diabetic in the south after living his entire childhood on a farm, after he left the south to live in city. He brought hard working hands that he was confident he could get him a job, working hard for his dreams. He had been told that he was "born to work" as a boy. There were many good seasons and a lot of work for him on the farm. Good seasons growing country crops, raising chickens, plowing the fields, with the amber red horse and blonde tail horse, and the mules, feeding, killing hogs, fishing in the farm lake, picking baskets full of apples and pears from the orchard, the corn, the string beans, Crowder peas, black berries, cherries trees, corn fields to get to, to get along, and bring up with the harvest at his father's farm during the summer. His father's only source of providing for the family. The farm was faithful with good produce, and a variety of foods to eat, that gave him energy and strength he would become known for on every job he undertook, all his life. On the farm there was a bounty of good food for the animals to be fed, fattened up. It eased the heavy feeling of carrying the knowledge of his purpose for being born, told him by his father. "Born to work". So he was a dutiful son and did what he was told, as a good buddy, born to work. This working hard he carried with him to the big city. As a young married father worked, worked hard. There was plenty good food to eat at his house. Even cherries, pecans, fish, was brought up for his young children to eat good like he did in the county all his life as boy. After all they grew all types of vegetables down south. Working so hard he made sure he had the good food, he ate with all his heart when he ate with his plate loaded up with delicious southern dishes. He never so no harm in eating all he wanted growing up. He worked off those pies, those pounds. He ate till he was full. He would never have dreamed he was eating too much. Good eating was a blessing from God to him. He deserved it, he earned it, he provided for him to have a good breakfast, lunch, and dinner like his mother cooked, and for his family. Then his thirst came, and all the symptoms. It was a blessing that he caught it, before he had a heart attack from the way was eating. would do more than testing his strength. But this strong man, a strong father never let anything move him. He worked hard at doing what his doctor told him. He changed his eating habits, by eating less of the same foods, until he couldn't eat them anymore without damaging his hart and his whole body. Soon he had his routine, his diet was right for his diabetes, and he went on working. Working hard. His mind was strong, his hands were strong, and his back was still strong like a mountain. He had will to survive his diabetes. But he was a man. He had the free will to choose, to choose to do what men do, drink and smoke, as he always did with his home cook meals. He liked to drink and smoke as much as he liked to eat. When he was done with his day's work he smoked. He rolled his cigarettes sometimes. He had rolled his father's farm home grown tobacco. Then he drank as a tradition with his father his brothers in the summer back down south for his vacation with his family. They men all met outside the town's old country hotel, next to the country liquor store, on the lot, where the country road stretched out in front of the store. The lot also was part of a dirt road. There on this rocky dirt road of the store lot, all the men stood, in a circle. They stood in a big circle and passed around a bottle of whiskey. Nothing but hard liquor for these men. Each took a drink from the same bottle. This how it was for years, the best whiskey. They were men. Men who worked hard and drank hard. And they could hold their liquor. Who would have thought this is where the diabetic heart began for this large family of big men and women, their sisters who were big like they were?

Drinking In The Circle Of Sons Of The Grandpa Who Sleep ON The Up Against The Wheel of His Truck

They were proud to smoke, proud to drink, and ready to eat a big meal while they continued to drink at the kitchen table. They loved to eat too. They loved good soul food cooking. The young, country, sun burnt skin father, a handsome black man, was not yet a father then. His hard work made him a stronger sports man. He loved sports with all his heart too. Even then he knew he'd work hard for the scouts that promised to come back for him, they saw he could swing a stick, he could catch, run and pitch and play any position in his favorite game. When they didn't come for him didn't matter, he go to them. He was raised on the best food for strength. He dreamed of having the best life God intended for him to live. He even saw across all the finest people in a local fair, a young beauty and knowing about her family he knew she would be a good mate. He made to the city, come to play ball, rejected at the gate, he went on his way. Went back, eloped with his country beautiful girl, a teen bride, who said, she dream of being a good wife, being a good mother, having children all her life. By twenty six they had five of them. Today would have never happened her starting as a teen child bride. He settled for his dream of a family, her good southern cooking, after he taught her with southern hospitality the art of southern cooking for the soul. As a child his mother sowed cooking lessons into his soul. Said he might be alone someday, so in just in case, a man needs to know. Mother knew the heart needs food to strengthen his soul. Who knew, from the southern kitchen, there would come a tremendous lesson? A new 65 Chevy off the rack, a running banged up 52 Chevy truck to haul loads of red bricks, tools and a lunch box full of soul food. Plants of wood piled up, to the Lord, the young father had much to give Thanks. He kept his cold glass of ice water that he couldn't work without. Crackers, thick slices of cheddar cheese, pickles, and hog head cheese, salami, bologna, were an option that became a working man's quick noontime delight. Rattling truck, wind skipping along on his arm out the driver's side, window. He never had a problem, not since that doctor diagnosed him at nineteen, of having diabetes. His children saw him and their young mother in love, kiss, and hug her, snug in his lap. He stood tall and his eyes laughed as if to say, see! Did you see that! He never once talked about the battle he fought with diabetes. He was a father, he was happy. His family ate together. This was a southern tradition, American eating, praying over their food, a united family is a blessing forever. But the big oval shaped plate he now ate from, piled with fried chicken, with his favorite, pinto beans, began to disagree with him. He ate the skin on the chicken, the kiss of death for a diabetic like him, in spite of him being a working man. Needless to say hard whisky didn't help him to listen. Gin didn't help, didn't balance the sugar. Sugar was the real problem even back then. Most everything he ate, drank, brought weight, pounds, too many calories* to his 6'3" height to 295lbs of muscle, he ate food that stuck to the ribs. He trusted southern wisdom, made his own ice cream. A man is not made of stone he is flesh and blood marrow and bones. His children and his wife loved to see the sight of him eating all that food that was what a hardworking man was supposed to do. He loved chumping down on raw white onions. He took every challenge like a man, that's what men do. That's what he believed, that that's what men do. His wife began to boil and bake his chicken, she would listen for him until he learned to listen. She loved him and was concerned for him, concerned for his heart. He was a diabetic 50 years. With her help the first twenty-five years he took good care of himself. His feet's history took him back to the black concrete roads, dirt roads, rock roads, in Mississippi, with him walking bare feet on hot surfaces, carrying his only pair of shoes, strolling in the heat. He lived the years of the depression era in the country, in America. He would be self-taught after 50 years later. He taught himself to read and write is his big chair, given to him by his closest brother. Enduring the worst life brought became a way of life on a machinist job, where his skills impressed, and sooth hard hearted hearts of men who looked at him as their enemy, they called a man a boy, boy do that!! Boy!!! Do this. Nothing could shake him. They could never make him leave. He was the last when all of them had passed. He out lasted all of them. He out lived them. He suffered because of them. He began to drink heavily because of them. But he was just being a man, that way. It was all he knew. The way a man has to. He was man enough to forgive them too. He took peace of mind home and his self-respect, intact, along with his retirement plaque* he would for the rest of his life, so prize. He was a diabetic even then, had all his children while he was yet a diabetic. A working man, he endured, overcame, and lived through all the humiliation, the shame, a voting man, during these years, his family never went hungry. He was a good provider, a storyteller. He loved a joke, serious humor. He'd called the person who told them a good liar. Even when somebody joked with him. He lived along with his wife and children, through Civil Rights and that included the marches, the Kennedy's assassination, all the time keeping his feelings inside single stated expressions like, "He was tough." Martin's view in the greatest speech he ever gave, thus father ever knew. He was smoothest with people because his love of muzic made him mellow, relax, country back cowboy suave. Muzic was on, in his house, his home, all along this journey. His heart was full of good harmonies, the Blues, and Jazz's greatest tunes. He knew he'd made a home to come home for his family. He introduced you to the crooning of a classic at Christmas, he loved Nat Kong Cole. He first fell in love with his wife, to *Unforgettable* by Nat King Cole. His romantic, sentimental wife. They did alright. And he let you know, sure, he was a diabetic, but *he* did alright. He never, throughout all those years, did he mention the term "diabetic heart". Being a diabetic 50 had years doesn't shake a man, a man has heart.

The Devil Is A Lying Spirit In The Smoke God Will Smoke Him Out

Dealing With Thickening Of The Vessels

It was going to a long road to beating smoking and drinking even though he was a diabetic. A drunk driver, a cigarette accident almost putting his son's eye out would become motivation, and ultimatums to quit. And he did. Drunkenness had a much worst end in store he didn't consider, the matter was biblical, he was blessed to have quit. But he always had hope of driving his Lincoln Continental again. He had done well for years on his own. Then the years were there where he began to depend on his children. Everybody, somebody needed to help him. Some complained about having the time, but they grew to enjoy helping him. They remembered how good he had been to them. Many of them had also learned to forgive him the drunken nights, years before that were followed by mornings of waking up to his regretful calling to wake his innocent victims, when he again was using that voice that that showed the good side of him, so he would be liked again. His children had left home years ago. God, little did he know, had spoken to his second son, who didn't know, he was the prodigal one, and told him in a dream, saying three times, "You need to go home." The one that didn't want to be like him. The gifted son that loved to read, was born an artist. But the son attributed his love of laying paint on, to his father who first taught him to be a painter, painting school walks. The letter he'd sent him revealed what he'd always been wondering about his father's love for him, his father's writing was at a third grade level, and that writing him took humbling his manly pride. God had his eye on him. There had to be a reason why God sent his son home. He was happy to see his son, to his son's surprise, and his son was happy to him, and to see his father who was a diabetic, doing well, and by God's grace they were both still alive. There was a chance to find healing. The total 25 years the son was traveling, moving, living, he brought back with him. The son planned to stay 30 days and return to the west coast. With his father looking well, smiling, he only wondered about why his father always had a pot of cabbage boiling on the stove. That was different. The Lincoln in the back yard out of commission was still working. The father was still taking care of himself. The father didn't need him as usual. Plus, he had all his other children. Even if they only occasionally came to see him. But within a short time the father became deftly ill. For as the cotton mouth goes unnoticed though

its head stuck out the murky water with crystal clear reflections of blue sky and jagged branches on the clear surface of a creek. Water that looks good, looks good for country boy's souls, who are familiar with red clay colored water in mud holes, and gold and green, wild creeks, and dives in believing what they see, and gets bitten by surprise. So can such appearance be on the surface, like it can be for an infected callous sore, hiding the infection, deeper under the hardened callous surface, on the diabetic's foot, that goes noticed. He was a good father, who, for the first 35 years as a diabetic did well on his own. Fifty years with a diabetic heart he was doing well after all those years, and looked good. His face was not wrinkled for his age. His back was clear, for the present, as his helpers could see, as he got cleaned up. He liked to put a new fresh outfit on. It was always easy, he had to be lifted up into his favorite chair. His smile was something to see. He sipped smoking umber brown, black coffee. He had been up, a sporadic shirt night's sleep didn't faze him, any more than anything that came his way. He was able to endure all he suffered through daily because he'd made up his mind the moment he accepted that diabetes came with the current conditions of his body. He was home, he lived with it. Technology was catching up to diabetes it seemed. Still, him being on all those pills, didn't sit well with his prodigal son who had come home after not seeing him for over decade, had stayed, because he realized, who was going to help him, when he got sick, shortly after his son came back. His son decided he'd stay a little longer, and a few months went by, then a year, two years, five years, seven years, ten years until the fifteenth year, the son was still there, caring for him in the way he did everything, with all his heart, to perfection. But perfection could not cure the father's diabetes, nor 27 pills a day, free nurses visits, checking up on him, doctor's visits, care giver after care giver, all different types, kinds of people from many different cultures, and places, some even ex-drug addicts who were clean, who got satisfaction from caring for the sick and got their humanity back that drugs took from them. All this comforted him, comfort his mind. All of this helped him. How many times did the flashing lights roll across the front of the flat top he owned, his home, and paid for, his place since the seventies? The very same type of flat top building that he worked on in the 1950s, when black people were not even allowed on this part of the Southside of the city. But here he was, and now he was the owner of the house he was denied even looking at. He'd come to the city for sports but end up at peace with be a dreamer about that. His dream to play baseball lived out through his three sons. His daughter even became all around highest trophy, winning, athlete. A competitor, in everything she did. She took care of things for him. He had it good because of her being such a smart disciplined approach to money, business, and being charming when she needed to be. The time she had was limited because of her being in demand on her job, as a seasoned expert in real estate related business. The father needed more help than being taken to checkups at the doctor, by ambulance. The many good years as a diabetic he expected would one day come to be the diabetic experience of his present life. The quality of his life hadn't changed much in his mind, but the father now had had both legs amputated. He was blessed to not have to work anymore, he had a pension, social security, and free services, medical, and medicine taken care of, and he was still doing well. The diabetes had caused him to lose his toe, then toes, foot and then feet and legs. He told his son he could eat anything but just in small amounts, he needed a little bit of fat, a glass of juice, to go with the meals he got delivered to him daily. So many benefits of free services he qualified for, dwindled before his son's eyes. Until they were all gone. Soon his son, who worked 40 hours, went to the university to finish college, also cared for him seven nights a week. Secretly, one day the son made a vow to care for father for the rest of his life, to sacrifice all his dreams, and just take care of the father. To comfort him as he looked at how sad his father's expression on his face had become. He took out his drawing paper, a large piece, and told his father, sit up, I want to do a painting of you. In just two hours he completed the painting. His father gave it that man's stern look he gave, as if judging the painting his son did, the way he did when he first taught him how to paint walls when he was a boy. His son hung the painting in a thick artist cardboard frame over the sealed chimney shelf in his father's bedroom. His father smiled. The painting was a great comfort to the father, it meant he and his son could get along, the past has been forgiven, they were friends after so many years of anger, gate and conflict. The son suddenly understood all the mood swings that came with diabetes, the fear, the depression, pain. There were things his father never explained about sugar, how drinking made his so bad, warp, why it had killed nearly all his fourteen siblings, and family members for years. None of his own children had become diabetics. It hit some of the grandchildren in their teens and twenties. He had been a diabetic 50 years and after the Million-man March 911, he saw the first black man running for

President, Barack Obama. He never dreamed he'd see it, but the son knew he was a dreamer. He always been a dreamer his whole life. His father lived to see him. His father always had this confidence, as if to say, I always said we would have one, a black man who could win, become the President. The father had become more disabled from being independent, to do things himself, as his pills, his medicines, medicines began to cripple his movement. Suddenly he could not put a spoon to his mouth. Months later this side effect was explained, when the son read the printout about the medicine. It that warned of this side effect). Medicine, all those pills, had taken its toll, his kidneys even went down into the teen percentages. Dialysis he'd promised himself, which took away all the beauty from his sister, he would not do. Even though her spirit remained as lively and vibrant as ever, the way she looked after troubled his heart. It was certain for him; it was something he would never do. She called him often to show how well she was able to live with what dialysis and diabetes had done to her. He refused dialysis, the day had come. He went home. His son wondered why he had never gone home to his hometown he loved so much. To the giant turtle of Tupelo. To his father's house and farm. He still owned land there. No the Tupelo he knew was gone. Like the old medicine treatment to heal was replaced with the new Silva dine patch, that healed the sore that covered his whole back, (that took a year of changing the bandages to heal), the healing from the old ways, what it could do was gone. Or so it seemed. No the father went home to his own bed. By refusing dialysis he had made his choice. His son slept in the joining front room. The Spirit woke his son. A small voice said, "Go check on Dad." When he went to. Look at his father. He asked, "Are you ok?" But father lay there. He murmured, "Yeah." He had made the choice to die. He didn't have to die at moment in his life. The dying stop speaking at that moment. The son stood over him. The son saw him cringe slightly. His son watched him take his past breath. The last fire truck arrived. They hooked him up to charge and shocked him back to life. His heart had stopped. The wait began after the coroner was called. The son stayed with him, standing at his bedside.

His body was still warm. The son never dreamed that years later he would be a diabetic too. But in the seven years that past the father could not have imagined the technological advances in medicine would give new knowledge into the cure for diabetes for his son. The years of caring for his diabetic father were healing years that went with his son, memories, lessons, wisdom, caring for his father that came to be a comfort to his heart, when he faced the family's affliction in a battle that went on for generations of his family. His father did not read or write to learn about advances in ways to care for, and meet, the challenges of diabetes. His father would have had to hear about fasting as a cure, his son who searched for years for a cure after he turned diabetic, did the search in the new generation of smart online. Combining less intrusive surgeries and plant based meals would have radically changed his father's life if he'd lived to the present time. Apple cider vinegar could have helped to keep his feet healthy, Reversing nerve damage. Herbal healing and improvement for circulation for vessels, natural antibiotics alternatives, the new knowledge about diabetes, healing. The father would not have looked on YouTube, or anywhere online to form an equation. The cure for diabetes is not in pills, not in insulin if insulin produces and causes the disease and the reactions in the problems that are the dual activities that formed the diabetic's life with diabetes. * The new approach might have saved the father from blowing out his kidneys with insulin. The use of spices to control and balance sugar might have been the better choice for a life without insulin. The most important benefits might have been freedom from medicines, which became such a comfort for the son who lives on, only now, knowing that there is hope, a cure, and considering his own diabetic lifestyle without depending on pills as a cure, knowing many such medicines is not the cure though they help for a time. Most important comforting the diabetic heart does not come from medicine but comes from living your full life, all of your experiences are what truly help. Your family, friends, people who take care of you, organ foods, the small meals, low calories, spices, your dreams, work, prayer all these things help. Many stories of diabetics dying in their sleep led the son to search for the most important solutions to the effects of diabetes on the different parts of the diabetic's body, especially the diabetic heart that can be harmed and hurt by diabetes the disease and sugar imbalances. God had already put the answers in nature as usual we were simply to discover them. The son quickly realized the answers parallel with such advanced and ancient practices of such basic things as fasting and using spices. Comforting the diabetic heart is separate to the challenge of the two parts of the diabetic's daily scare focused on the insulin disease and sugar imbalance health battle of diabetes. Natural ways to heal are best, not medicine that he was prescribes and had taking for a short time compared to those who now were dependent more so, after taking the shots, pills, for a longer time like past and many current type 2 the son like his self-care and care. The son, like his father was not a type 1 diabetic. But like his 13 year old nephew and 21 year old nephew, he had reach the point of managing the cure, the lifestyle, by fasting (with red grapes to snack on) to keep his sugar from dropping too low, eating an apple between meals for sugar balance, drinking red grape fruit juice for the liver, taking a spoonful of olive oil for the liver, buying a stack of bags of celery for his kidneys, taking baking soda, once a month, to clean his kidneys, (watching out for high blood pressure it caused him once, when he took too much, eating his favorite mixed nuts, (walnuts, almonds and pumpkin seed mixture), cooking his father's *Salmon Croquette* recipe with his spices, and turmeric, garlic, and onions. He had come a long way since that day he is sugar was at 752, when he learned that at 500 he should have been un a coma. He assessed he could have been dying at that moment, he did see people walking through the air, and he did hear a voice say, "Why don't you call an ambulance." And he did, making it into an emergency room bed where they couldn't even get his sugar to come down and he was on 30 minute watched all night, with his sugar being checked every 15 minutes. He was told that night he would now be diabetic for the rest of his life. His heart entered into a heaviness at that moment. He felt heart broken, he had searched for a cure since he was 19 for diabetes and Alzheimer's, fortunately he had been the one person who had never had a sugar problem he always prided himself for accomplishing. He attributed it to being an herbalist, eating vegetarian a lot, but he never suspected juices and never thought about *additives* as being causes for generational diseases. he by right eating and exercise discontinued his dependence on insulin. The comforting of the diabetic heart came from being loved by somebody who cared and cared for him. He learned much from his father about how to deal with diabetes. The knowledge and experiences he gained from helping his father are still with him today. It taught him what was the way to comforting the diabetic heart was love. To know his father left a legacy that helped to end the missing knowledge of how to cure diabetes in his family was comforting to his son's heart, that his story when he looked back was a story that could be a comfort to many a diabetic heart.

www.ingramcontent.com/pod-product-compliance
Lightning Source LLC
Chambersburg PA
CBHW050703250726
48662CB00002B/821